Two Envelopes is not just another end-of-life planning workbook. It is a uniquely personal resource, like sitting at the kitchen table with a dear friend sharing coffee and conversation about hard decisions. The steps are practical and uncomplicated, yet when completed, the *Two Envelope* plan will provide your family members a clear and concise way to recognize and honor your late-life decisions. Most of all, *Two Envelopes* offers an opportunity to give peace of mind and comfort to your dearest loved ones in a season that is riddled with deep grief and uncertainty.

Missy Buchanan, best-selling author of many books on faith and aging

Two Envelopes is so informative and full of useful information for families going through the most difficult times in their lives. Rusty offers such knowledge and wisdom in guiding people through the process of pre-planning. As a funeral professional, I work with families every day as they plan for the inevitable. Rusty captures the most important aspects of this extremely difficult and emotional time. I truly believe that everyone could benefit from following the guide that she has provided.

Joshua Tobias, Director of The Ira Kaufman Chapel, Southfield, Michigan

As Rusty Rosman shows us, it is never too soon to gather our loved ones and pose the hard questions that will ensure our wishes are honored both in life and in death. With deep gratitude to Rusty, we have her exceptionally comprehensive book, giving us the permission to gather with loved ones and have productive conversations we all need to share.

Rabbi Joseph Krakoff, CEO of the Jewish Hospice and Chaplaincy Network

Many families believe they've prepared for the end of life by making arrangements for funerals or safeguarding assets with legal counsel. Yet, they often overlook so many crucial details that truly matter. ... This book adeptly guides families through the necessary conversations and offers insights into how to approach these decisions with sensitivity and effectiveness. Rusty Rosman, with immense love and care, not only navigated these challenging discussions within her own family, but also lent her guidance to countless friends and relatives over many years. She meticulously crafted this book to ensure that others don't have to embark on this journey blindly.
Lauren Rosman O'Desky, Owner of Oasis Senior Advisors and WellSpring Care Management

We are all going to die. *Two Envelopes* will bring you peace of mind because it sets clear and concise directions for you to consider and write about for your family and loved ones. By putting your instructions on paper in these envelopes, you will find comfort and satisfaction for your end of life wishes. It did for me—and I know it will for you.
Joanne Rosenthal Goldstein, Rusty's sister who shares the family wisdom readers will find in *Two Envelopes*

A must read for every senior! An excellent way to share the most important information with your family. The author is very insightful on the needs of families. This book is an incredible gift to/for your family.
Ida Goutman, CEO Cruz Clinic Psychiatric and Psychological Care

My mother was diagnosed with a terminal illness. During this stressful and confusing time, the guidance set out in what was then a draft of *Two Envelopes* helped ground and organize my mother. She focused on what she wanted to do as outlined in this book and then proceeded to do it. She felt she had a measure of control in a situation that afforded her little control. Our family was so grateful to have this guide. *Two Envelopes* gave all of us comfort and peace of mind.
Elizabeth Sandler, a daughter of an early user of *Two Envelopes*

Two Envelopes is a how-to guide for peace of mind. It provides thoughtful steps for important too-often postponed decisions and how to share them effectively with family and others. It shows each of us how a simple envelope can be transformed into a meaningful vessel of love.
Margo Gold, Rusty's sister, community activist and volunteer in Atlanta

I read *Two Envelopes* both as an attorney from a professional view as well as an individual in all the various perspectives that one might find themselves, be it a father, husband, child, grandfather. This book will appeal to everyone irrespective of ethnicity, social, economic or educational background. *Two Envelopes* helps readers consider complicated and sensitive issues that they may encounter while planning for their later years. It accomplishes these goals with suggestions drawn from personal insight, foresight, compassion, logic and understanding.

Two Envelopes becomes a source of reliance, and therefore comfort, even in the most difficult of family situations. Rusty Rosman helps all of us to objectively identify our concerns and hopes for our loved ones. This is an outstanding resource for all. I am sure that the parents to whom this book is dedicated would have been so very proud.
Donald Wagner, an early reviewer of *Two Envelopes*

Two Envelopes

What You Want Your Loved
Ones To Know When You Die

Rusty Rosman

Copyright © 2024 by Barbara Gayle Rosman

All rights reserved.

ISBN: 978-1-64180-175-1

Version 1.0

Cover design by Rick Nease
RickNeaseArt.com

Published by
Front Edge Publishing, LLC
42807 Ford Road, No. 234
Canton, MI, 48187

Front Edge Publishing books are available for discount bulk purchases for events, corporate use and small groups. Special editions, including books with corporate logos, personalized covers and customized interiors are available for purchase. For more information, contact Front Edge Publishing at info@FrontEdgePublishing.com.

Disclaimer: The information, advice and recommendations provided in this book are not, nor are they intended to be, a substitute for legal advice or financial advice. Legal advice should be sought and obtained from a licensed attorney. Financial advice should be sought and obtained from a licensed/certified accountant and/or financial advisor. Always seek professional legal and financial advice when preparing your estate for your eventual passing.

Dedicated with love to my parents, of blessed memory,
Dorothy and Jay Rosenthal
who gave this gift of love to me and to my siblings.

Contents

Foreword by Missy Buchanan xiii
Preface by Rabbi Joseph H. Krakoff xvi
Introduction by Lauren Rosman O'Desky xviii

PART 1: Getting Started
   Preparing to Create Your Two Envelopes 1

PART 2: Envelope #1
   Your Funeral Arrangements 7
   All About You 12
   Personalizing Your Obituary, Death Notice and Eulogy 14
   Funeral and Burial 16
   Mourning and Grieving 20

PART 3: Envelope #2
   Preparing This Envelope 25
   Write a Love Letter 36
   And from Me to You 37
   What to Do with Your Two Envelopes 38

Acknowledgments 40
About the Author 42
Reach Out to Rusty 43
Notes for Your Two Envelopes 45

Foreword

As I write this foreword, I am knee deep in my own season of grief. My beloved husband died just a few months ago after a brief illness. I am a person of deep faith, but his unexpected death upended my world and shook me to the core. This intimate experience with death also makes the wisdom of *Two Envelopes* especially relevant for me in real time.

My husband and I had been proactive in planning for our late lives. We had already downsized to a smaller, single-level home and simplified our belongings. We had updated legal and financial documents and pre-purchased funeral home arrangements. We had penned our life stories, including photos, as a gift to our children and grandchildren. We had created a photo book of family keepsakes along with the history of each item. As a long-married couple and the parents of three adult children, we were confident we had completed the important work of preparing for late life and death. Yet, once my husband died, I soon realized how much more we could have done to make this journey less stressful for our family as we tried to navigate both the practical and emotional aftershocks of death.

On the afternoon my two oldest children and I left the funeral home following my husband's death, they hugged me in the parking lot and offered authentic words of thanks. Through their tears, it was evident they had a new appreciation for the preparations my husband and I had made regarding our late lives and eventual deaths. For the first time, they understood it was our gift to them and their sister. In fact, the only decision we had to make that day at the funeral home was which seasonal flowers to include in the arrangements for the church service.

When we returned home, though, we discovered some unexpected challenges looming over us. We searched for and found the red folder of passwords for my husband's digital devices but learned that some passwords had not been updated. We soon realized that his primary email, associated with his real estate business, was set to be dismantled in a few days, leaving us to scramble to identify which online accounts, including automatic payments, were associated with his email address so that we could change the accounts to my email address. Even as we were selecting the photographs and the music for his Celebration of Life service, we were working to determine if our insurance autopayment was charged to one of our credit cards or if it was drafted from a checking account.

Grief felt like a stressful tug-of-war between practical tasks and the emotional toll of an overwhelming loss.

As a writer-speaker on issues of aging and faith and an older-adult-ministry volunteer, I was already familiar with many of the challenges that come with the end of life. I have held the hands of many older adults, including my own parents, and listened to their concerns in their final days. I have counseled adult children as they struggled to discern their parent's unvoiced thoughts about cremation or burial. Regrettably, I also have seen adult children squabble about the wording of an obituary while their dying loved one rested nearby in a drug-induced fog. I have known siblings who insisted on two separate memorial services for their mother because they could not agree on their loved one's wishes.

When speaking to groups of adult children and aging parents, I encourage both generations to initiate important end-of-life conversations. Many are resistant, though, and plug their ears with their fingers, saying it's just too depressing. They fail to see the truth:

The most depressing thing is the chaos that follows when preparations have been left undone.

Two Envelopes is not just another end-of-life planning workbook. It is a uniquely personal resource, like sitting at the kitchen table with a dear friend sharing coffee and conversation about hard decisions. The steps are practical and uncomplicated, yet when completed, the *Two Envelope* plan will provide your family members a clear and concise way to recognize and honor your late-life decisions. Most of all, *Two Envelopes* offers an opportunity to give peace of mind and comfort to your dearest loved ones in a season that is riddled with deep grief and uncertainty.

Missy Buchanan is the best-selling author of many books about aging and faith. She has been featured on *Good Morning America* with co-anchor Robin Roberts because Missy was chosen by Robin's mother Lucimarian Roberts to help them write their mother-daughter memoir, *My Story, My Song*.

Preface

Among the most difficult conversations amongst loved ones is to talk about anything having to do with our death. No one wants to confront their own mortality and to think that there will be a day that they are no longer walking this earth.

When we are young, we presume that we will live forever—whatever that means. And as we get older, while we realize that this is definitely not in the cards, it is still a topic that does not easily cross our lips.

I think back to the births of my three children. They were among the happiest days of my life—as was my wedding! And I will never forget how impossibly difficult it was for my wife and I to sit opposite our estate planner when our children were quite young as he bid us to think about what would happen—God forbid—if we should die before our kids reached adulthood. The lawyer took us on a mind-boggling journey beyond this world—a place we didn't want to even visit for a moment. And this is not an unusual response in our society even though death is wholly inevitable.

One of the most touching and emotional scenes in the entire Bible is when Jacob is dying and summons his children to the deathbed. As it says in Genesis 49:33: "When Jacob finished instructing his sons, he drew his feet into the bed and, breathing his last, he was gathered to his people." I imagine that in those final moments of life Jacob is giving his progeny the details they need to fulfill some of his final wishes—funeral, eulogy, burial, etc.

While I am grateful that the Torah transmits this scene to us, I admit I struggle with the idea that Jacob waited until merely moments before his demise to gather his children together to have this conversation. I feel badly that Jacob never found the opportunity before that point to share with his children the equivalent of an advanced directive or an ethical will.

As a rabbi who specializes in hospice work, I am regularly having end-of-life conversations with patients and their families, often for the first time just hours before they pass. What I find time and again is that individuals have rarely made their wishes known because thinking about the end was just too painful to bear. I get that. I really do! But, as hard as these conversations are to conjure, they are essential to giving the surviving family members the peace of mind to know that they are doing everything possible to honor the wishes of their loved one.

Perhaps we wait so long because we don't know how to get started or we don't know what the proper questions are to ask. Well now we do!

With deep gratitude to Rusty Rosman, we have her exceptionally comprehensive *Two Envelopes*, giving us the permission to gather with loved ones and have productive conversations around end-of-life questions. As Rusty shows us, it is never too soon to gather our loved ones and pose the hard questions that will ensure our wishes are honored both in life and in death.

Life is short and truthfully—we never know what will happen tomorrow. It is a gift that keeps on giving to make our decisions today and not have to rely on others who think they are doing what we would have wanted.

Thank you, Rusty for giving us this inspiring guidebook that will help us help each other now—as well as from generation to generation. May we all go from strength to strength.

Rabbi Joseph H. Krakoff is CEO of The Jewish Hospice and Chaplaincy Network (JHCH), based in West Bloomfield, Michigan, and author of *Never Long Enough: Finding comfort and hope amidst grief and loss*.

Introduction

Throughout my life, I've had the privilege of witnessing my mother, the distinguished author of this book, serve as an unwavering advocate, compassionate guide and dedicated caretaker.

Her journey as a caregiver began with her own parents as she provided support through various phases of their lives: from homecare to assisted living, and ultimately, nursing home care. She extended her compassion to her mother-in-law, even amidst a less-than-warm relationship, persevering through the same continuum of care. Her dedication didn't stop there; she reached out to help numerous friends, young and old, who found themselves navigating this challenging path alone.

In my capacity as a Certified Senior Advisor—and as the owner of multiple businesses specializing in senior care, including geriatric care management, consulting and placement services—I can confidently attest that this book is a treasure not only for yourself but also for your entire family.

Two Envelopes is a gift that may come as a revelation. Many families believe they've prepared for the end of life by making arrangements for funerals or safeguarding assets with legal counsel. Yet, they often overlook the crucial details that truly matter. It's rare for families to dispute the color of a casket or the inscription on a headstone. Instead, they grapple with Mom's treasured ring or Dad's unspoken wishes after a stroke. These disputes often revolve around matters of money and power. This book adeptly guides families through the necessary conversations and offers insights into how to approach them with sensitivity and effectiveness.

With immense love and care, my mother not only navigated these challenging discussions within her own family but also lent her guidance to countless friends and relatives over many years. She meticulously crafted this book to ensure that others don't have to embark on this journey blindly.

In my professional life, I frequently find myself engaging in conversations that many shy away from. There's no denying it—it's a daunting task. That's why *Two Envelopes* will be such an indispensable roadmap for families. This book not only illuminates the critical considerations surrounding health and end-of-life matters for you, your loved ones or your friends but also provides a blueprint for addressing each topic with empathy, compassion and diplomacy.

I implore you to do yourself and your family a favor by delving into the pages of this book and completing the journey it outlines. The legacy you leave behind in this world is often shaped by how others remember you once you've passed.

While caring for someone by being present and providing for their needs is a noble endeavor, demonstrating the forethought and care to ease the transition after your own passing is an immeasurable gift. *Two Envelopes* eloquently encapsulates the essence of this profound and enduring gift.

Lauren Rosman O'Desky, CSA, is the owner of Oasis Senior Advisors and WellSpring Care Management.

Getting Started

It's not always easy to think about dying—but each of us will, ready or not.

I wrote *Two Envelopes* to share what I have learned in helping my parents and countless others guide their loved ones with what to do after the death of a family member. Preparing Envelope #1 and Envelope #2 gives your family and those important to you the greatest gift of your love—telling them what to do after you die so they don't have to figure it out alone.

Tell your family what you want. They don't have to think about what you *would* want, and whether it is right or not—you are telling them. They want to do what you want. *Two Envelopes* helps you tell them.

> *I wish you peace of mind as you go through preparing your family for your death. Yes, you'll cry a lot. There are so many hard things to decide, and you will often question yourself as you prepare your envelopes. Throughout this preparation, remember how much you love your family and will do anything to make this time of their lives less stressful. This is the hardest thing you will ever do to make it easier for the ones you love the most. They will appreciate what you did for them and love you for it.*

I know this works. My dear friend died recently and, while my heart still hurts, I am comforted by what she said about Two Envelopes: "I did it!" She told me she had checked off, paragraph by paragraph, what she had completed. When we hugged goodbye just before she died, she told me that I gave her a huge gift: peace of mind. She helped write her obituary, chose the picture she wanted with her obituary, wrote out what she wanted done with her belongings, worked with her legal and financial advisors and, best of all, wrote a love letter to her children. I will always be grateful that while I couldn't make her well, I did give her the path to follow for peace of mind. I will always treasure our friendship and that I helped my dear friend be comforted.

I was going to enclose two envelopes for you, but I realized that you will be choosing how much you want to put in each envelope, as well as where you will put them for your family to reach for when it's time. So, I leave it to you to select the size of the envelope that is best for you. As time goes on, you may want to change the size of the envelopes and they may need to be placed in a different location than you originally thought.

Please keep in mind how important it is for you to date each page you place in your envelopes. You may choose to amend what you previously wrote or possibly discard papers. This way, you as well as those who read these pages, will know your most recent thoughts. Also, label your envelopes: "#1: Open Immediately After I Die" and "#2: Open Immediately After the Funeral." Now your loved ones know that you have carefully thought out what you want to happen after you die and what you want them to do.

There are a few important things to remember: Not everyone is blessed with a great family or, as time has gone by, has family. You may have a wonderful friend, a distant relative, a colleague, someone you consider your inner circle, or you have appointed a funeral representative or a trustee. I've written this from a family point of view but it's easy to read it as your inner circle instead of your spouse, family and children.

Each one of us has our own faith, culture and practices, handed down generation to generation. And, this book includes basic practices of different ethnic and religious beliefs. I have met with numerous religious leaders and funeral directors regarding religious and funeral practices. By no means is Two Envelopes a complete and binding way of conducting end of life rituals. Consider consulting with your religious leader about the practices you observe AND with the funeral home that honors your religious practices. Incorporate your beliefs and wishes into Envelope #1 and Envelope #2. This is so important for you and your family because it is familiar to you and comforting for your loved ones. I have written this book from my own Jewish experiences and each one of you can easily incorporate your own faith practices throughout the book.

We all know this to be true:
  We all die.
  We all mourn the passing of loved ones.
  We all must deal with the details related to our loved ones death.

Your family will appreciate you even more because of what you placed in your Two Envelopes.

Preparing to Create Your Two Envelopes

Your Two Envelopes contain your thoughts and wishes for your family after your death. It's important to think about and write down what is important to **you**—your beliefs and your family values and history. Hopefully, your attention to the details surrounding your death will help your children feel that they were able to follow your wishes.

Write on the outside of one envelope:

#1
Open Immediately After I Die

Envelope #1 will contain all the pertinent information your family will need for the visitation, funeral, burial and, in Jewish families, the shiva (visitation that follows burial). This envelope needs to be opened immediately after your death, because it contains information your family will use immediately.

Write on the outside of the other envelope:

#2
Open Immediately After the Funeral

Envelope #2 is ***not*** in place of a will or trust, which are legal documents. Envelope #2 contains ***your*** thoughts and directions for your loved ones outside of your will and trust.

Why envelopes?

Why envelopes and not a computer file? Because your loved ones can easily find envelopes. They may not know the current password to your computer, or you may not have created this in a computer file format that they can open.

As you do the hard work that's necessary to fill your envelopes, keep in mind that this entire exercise is about you and your inner circle, which could include others beyond just your children and spouse. Don't be afraid, though, to limit the conversation to those you truly consider part of that inner circle. It is important that everyone who is closest to you has the same understanding of who is to be involved in decision making and in what role.

Consider family dynamics

My mother used to tell me, "One mother can raise twelve children, but twelve children cannot agree how to take care of their one mother."

My mother was very wise.

Families are the most complicated entities on earth. In a perfect world, everyone in a family would love each other equally, get along perfectly, never be jealous of or angry with another family member—*if only!* But, as we all know, a perfect family doesn't exist. And death can bring out the best and the worst in family members.

It's not unusual for there to be differences of opinion on what to do and how to move forward following a death in the family. Your Two Envelopes will provide your family with clear instructions about how **you** want your final arrangements to be handled. If there is an area of contention in your family and you want to address it, this is the place to do it. Acknowledging this contention is difficult, but necessary. Think it out and write it out.

Two Envelopes will help you navigate the areas that are most likely to cause family discord and to make sure that your wishes are followed in the days and weeks after your death, hopefully mitigating some of the tension that might occur in the absence of your guidance and instructions.

We all know families come in different shapes and sizes. Some families are the ones we are born or adopted into, some have members that have been estranged for years, others are made up of friends, some are blended by marriage or consent.

So many different kinds of families!

Not everyone has children, a spouse or a significant other. You may have outlived your family members and now find yourself alone in your planning. As you read *Two Envelopes*, keep in mind that you may want to substitute the words "inner circle" or "loved ones" where I have used terms like "spouse," "family" or "children."

For those who are alone (but you're really not alone)—Life has many twists and turns. If you do not have a spouse, children or siblings, talk to your legal advisor about whom you should designate to handle your affairs after you die. Some people might choose to have a dear friend, others may feel more comfortable with a trustee or a legal representative. You should receive that person's permission to be the designated handler of your affairs and make that part of your will. Be sure that the designated person knows where to find your envelopes so your wishes will be carried out.

Blended families—Blended families have their own dynamics that need to be addressed in this process. In such a family, you may be working through not only complicated and sometimes sensitive relationships, but also a range of unique legal, financial and procedural dynamics. One of the most difficult decisions is where do you wish to be buried or have your ashes placed. Some may wish to be with the parent of their children or their current spouse. Take the time to consider what is best for you and your blended family. There's much to think about. Your legal, financial and spiritual advisors can serve as helpful resources as you determine how best to navigate these potentially complex waters.

Planning with a spouse or partner—It is not unusual if your spouse/partner does *not* want to talk about life after your death. While that's understandable, it's not fair to you and your family. This is the time to be diplomatic but very firm. You are half of this relationship, and their half doesn't have more sway in this matter than your half.

If you find consistent resistance from your spouse, remind them that making these decisions is important to you and important to your shared family. Tell your partner that you intend to make a decision on a given topic. Tell them they have sixty days to think about it and provide input—and tell them on the sixty-first day *you* will make the decision yourself. This is not easy, but it's necessary for your piece of mind and really, for theirs, too.

Two days before your announced deadline, they will say, "Fine, we can talk." I've seen this happen numerous times.

No one likes to be pushed to make a decision, but these are decisions you do want to make yourselves and not leave up to your family alone. There is a sense of relief each time you add something to your envelopes. You are beginning the process of helping your loved ones handle all the details following your death.

Envelope #1

Your Funeral Arrangements

After a loved one's death, we want guidance on what to do next. Most American families work with a funeral home for burial and cremation services. Assuming you have chosen a funeral home, the first thing your family should see in Envelope #1 is the name of the funeral home you wish to use. Spell out what arrangements you may previously have made.

Whatever faith your family follows, your end-of-life traditions may stretch back centuries. As you are preparing Envelope #1, reach out to your own clergy. Even if you have not been active in a congregation in recent years, your clergy are glad to talk with you about what to expect and work with you to plan your service.

This is the time to think about which funeral home you prefer. You may want to speak with your spiritual leader about what funeral home best reflects your preferences for either burial or cremation. Some may prefer to make their own arrangements with a cremation service. Choosing a funeral home in advance and even prepaying for funeral services is not unusual. Parents who choose to do this save their children from having to select a casket and other decisions. Funeral directors do this every day and find it is a huge comfort for the person making their own arrangements. Think about having the conversation with your funeral director of choice and learn if this is the right path for you.

If you have belonged to an organization such as a Masonic lodge, let the funeral home director know so they can arrange for whatever honors should be included with the funeral.

Families with no religious affiliation, or individuals who describe themselves as secular, humanist or atheist, also find that funeral directors can be very helpful at the end of life. Most have staff trained in a wide array of options—religious and nonreligious.

How will your family reach the people who are important to you?

Your children may not know who was in your life on a daily basis, who your friends from your past were, who your work colleagues were, or who else you would want them to notify with the news of your death.

- Write out the names of those you would like notified of your death, including relatives your age you may be in contact with who your children are not familiar with, friends who no longer live in your city, people you worked with, boards and organizations you are a part of, and other people who are important to you.
- Write out their U.S. mail addresses, their email addresses and phone numbers. Put a date on this list.
- Also include the names of any publications where you would like your death notice to appear. Your children may not know how important it is to you to have your death notice appear in a particular organization's newsletter or a regional publication.
- Share this list with the funeral home as well, because they often help to place death notices.

Burial arrangements

In the 21st century, we have seen a major change in American views on burial and cremation. In recent years, the majority of all death remains in the United States are cremated. If you choose cremation, discuss with your family or representative what you wish done with your cremains. Talk with your funeral director about what options there are for cremains. There are many rules for what is allowed and what is not allowed for the dispersal of cremains, and they can vary state to state.

This is the time to talk with your spouse and children if you want to be placed in a cemetery. Cemeteries offer many choices: burial plots, columbaria (a wall for cremation urns) and other options. *Buy those spaces now!* It's a very difficult conversation, no doubt about it, but it's even worse after a loved one dies and no plans are in place for burial. In today's world, where so many children do not live in the same state, let alone the same country as their parents, making these arrangements at the time of death becomes a huge burden and often causes contention between siblings.

This is the time for you to do your research on which cemetery best fits your wishes. Sometimes this is a hard decision because you may have parents who own plots possibly in different cemeteries or you live in a different city than your parents and your children. Some cemeteries don't allow for cremated remains, if that is your preferred interment method. Some Jewish cemeteries do not allow non-Jewish partners to be buried in all sections. Make appointments with the executive directors of the cemeteries you are interested in to learn about costs and care of the graves and any relevant restrictions.

Cremation

Many people are choosing cremation now. Do talk with your legal advisor, your clergy, your funeral director and cemetery of choice (if you want your remains buried) so you make an informed decision about what is allowed and what is legal in your state. It's possible not every family member will approve of your choice to be cremated, so be clear you have thought this out and put in place what you want.

- Designate who will receive your ashes.
- What do you want to have happen with your ashes? This could possibly be a contentious choice for your family.
- If you think this may be a contentious issue in your family, talk to your legal advisor about a funeral representative document.
- Be sure to include this information in Envelope #1.

Once you are ready to make a decision, get out the tissue box, sit down and talk to your family about which city and cemetery you prefer for interment. Do your children wish to have cemetery spaces with you?

Veterans

This is the time to find your veteran papers and include a copy of them in Envelope #1. Your funeral director will help your family be sure that all funeral honors you are entitled to will be included in your funeral service. Without these papers, your family cannot be sure you will receive veteran honors that would be bestowed upon you at your funeral or burial. If you do not know where your papers are, make the time to contact the Bureau of Veterans Affairs and find out what you need to do to procure your records. This could take a great deal of time, so do it now.

Designating memorial donations and flowers

Do you wish to designate memorial donations in your funeral notice? People may choose to make a donation, which is a beautiful way to perpetuate your memory. Do you have a named fund at an organization or institution? A favorite charity? A meaningful organization you support? Would you prefer to have the donor select a charity of their choice?

Family members may not be in agreement on where to have these donations directed. Your death—your choice. So, write down your directions for where you would like memorial donations to be directed.

In many religions and cultures, sending flowers to the funeral is very appropriate. Families do appreciate the loving notes that are included with the flowers. If you have a preference concerning flowers, be sure to put that in this envelope.

All About You

Your name

What name do you want people to use?

While it may seem obvious that your family would know your name, it's not always as easy as we think! Write out your entire name—the one you were born with, the married names you have and your nicknames. Write down what name you want used in your death notices, eulogy and grave marker. My legal name is Barbara, but I have been called "Rusty" from the day I was born.

Religious and cultural names

As a Jewish person, you were traditionally given a Hebrew/Yiddish name at birth. Your Hebrew name is used to name you at the bris/baby naming, your bar/bat mitzvah, your marriage and when you die. Your children may not know your Hebrew name. Your parents' Hebrew names are equally important because you are called son or daughter of your parents at all religious rituals and burial is a religious ritual.

If you don't know your parents' Hebrew names and you are married, look at your Jewish wedding certificate, your Ketubah. Your Hebrew names are on it and so are your parents' names. If you don't have a Ketubah and your parents are deceased, call the cemeteries where your parents are buried; they will have the Hebrew names in their records. If you cannot find the names easily, call the funeral home you want your family to use and share this with them. They will be able to guide you to a rabbi who could help you figure out Hebrew names based on what history you share with them.

Many religions and cultures have their own naming rituals. In Christian traditions, religious names sometimes are given at baptism or other milestone events. In addition, some cultures around the world have naming practices that include ancestors or other honorific phrases in the full version of your name. Write down what names you want clergy to use and what names you want in death notices.

Help your family to understand the names that matter to you. Do this now because you know more about your family's traditions than your children do and it's worth your time for everyone's peace of mind.

Pictures of you

Your family may want to make a memory board or slide show. You need to write down where to find your photos. Are they on your computer? Your phone? Albums? CDs? Also, provide a password if your photos are on your phone or computer.

4

Personalizing Your Obituary, Death Notice and Eulogy

It's important to understand that a death notice, obituary and eulogy are three separate entities. A death notice is a paid announcement of your death that funeral homes help the family write. This notice will be placed in publications your family designates. An obituary is an article about a person who has died that a newspaper or magazine staff may choose to write at no cost to your family. A eulogy is different. It's either a written or spoken tribute to a person who has died, often personalized by the person delivering the eulogy. Eulogies are given at the funeral or memorial service.

Help your loved ones tell your story.

Write down stories you would love to hear if you were at your own funeral. This will help those mourning you to remember wonderful moments and stories they may have forgotten—or perhaps never even knew were a part of your early life. This could become a treasured memory for your family.

Write down memories your survivors may not recall:

- List any family members or special friends you want named in the "survived by" section of your obituary or death notice.

- Choose a picture of yourself that you prefer for these notices. Find a good head-and-shoulders photograph of yourself alone. Perhaps you might want to take a new photo. If this is a digital photo, be sure that it is high resolution so your photo will reproduce well.
- Details of your birth, childhood and schooling.
- Any military service.
- Details of your employment, the names of companies or institutions where you worked, your titles and what you did in your work life.
- Volunteer work you enjoyed.
- Organizations that mattered to you.
- Awards and honors that were bestowed upon you.

Faced with providing information for a death notice, obituary or eulogy, your family will thank you for providing accurate details. This way you are ensuring that the most enduring public article about your life is accurate.

Memorial donations

People may choose to make a donation to honor your memory rather than send flowers. Do you have a named fund at an organization or institution? A favorite charity? A meaningful organization you support? Would you prefer to have the donor select a charity of their choice? Family members may not be in agreement on where to have the donations directed so making these decisions now will make sure your choices will be honored. This is important for funeral information.

- Write down your directions for where you would like memorial donations to be directed.

5

Funeral and Burial

Funeral customs can be varied and yet similar. Every religion has its own funeral customs and they bring comfort to those who are mourning. There is a service, there is clergy, there are prayers and there is a meal following the burial or service. It's important and comforting for the family and friends that there is an order to grieving.

There is a distinct difference between the terms funeral and memorial service. At a funeral, the body is present in a casket. At a memorial service, there isn't a body or casket; instead a picture and/or an urn of the ashes is present.

Many religions have the visitation and funeral at the funeral home. Some religions' customs have the visitation at the funeral home and the funeral at the church. Some religions don't have visitation at all, just the funeral at the funeral home. Visitation (which could be called a wake) days have their own culture. The casket is always open. Discuss with your family how many days of visitation you want them to have. Family members of the deceased are present during several days of visitation. In today's world, visitation has frequently been scaled down to a day or two and one evening of visitation with a prayer service often during the evening visitation. Because of staffing issues, many cemeteries have set time for a casket to arrive and burial to begin, so the timing of funerals has become a necessity. Funeral directors are well versed in all the customs and regulations for funerals, cremation and burial so consult with them while doing your thinking and writing. The more thinking and writing you do, the easier it is for your loved ones to attend to your last wishes. If you have a definite opinion of what you want for your funeral, this is the place to be very specific. Remember, this is your opportunity to tell your family what you want and how you want your funeral arrangements to be handled. Think it out and write it down.

The funeral

These funeral practices have been shared with me by several funeral directors. Each region of the country and world has its own take on religious customs, so use the following as a guide and then customize your plans to what is familiar and comfortable to you.

Each religion has its own customs and practices regarding death. As the years have gone by, many customs and practices have been modified because of cultural changes, distance between families and beloved places of worship that are no longer in existence. It is important that you tell your family which customs and practices you want them to observe. Put it in writing so they will know what you want.

Catholic

Visitation/viewing is an important part of the Catholic funeral process. This occurs at the funeral home for an amount of time prior to the day of the funeral. Considering a person's age and the age of their friends and colleagues who will come to the visitation, give your family permission to choose how many days of visitation there should be. A prayer service is often part of the evening visitation hours.

A funeral mass is part of a Catholic funeral and takes place in the church. There will often be a rosary service. Because so many

Catholic churches have closed in recent years, give your family/representative permission to select another priest or church if yours has closed since you created this part of Envelope #1.

After the Catholic funeral and burial, there is a memorial meal. It can be at the church, a rental hall or in a restaurant.

Christian

There are multiple denominations of Christianity. It's best to check with your clergy as to your practices and write them down so your family can inform the funeral home. Many of the funerals of people of Christian faiths occur at a funeral home. Visitation is traditionally part of a funeral and takes place at the funeral home. If the family desires, the funeral can take place at the church. There is a meal after the funeral or burial to which those in attendance are invited. The meal is often called a memorial meal and can be at a banquet hall, a restaurant or at the church.

Greek Orthodox

Visitation is at the funeral home and all Greek Orthodox funerals are in the church. The Greek Orthodox tradition does not cremate; they exclusively choose burial. The meal after the burial is called the mercy meal. Forty days after burial, the Trisagion service takes place in the church.

Muslim

The funeral and burial all happen within one day. The funeral begins at the funeral home, where the family assists with washing the body and preparing it for burial. Then the family accompanies the casket to the mosque. There is a viewing hour and then the imam leads the prayer for the dead, called Janazah. Burial follows immediately after the service is concluded. Many cemeteries have a Muslim section. There is a funeral meal after the burial at the cemetery. The condolences visitation and prayers at the mosque often take place a week after burial.

African American

The public/viewing visitation takes place at the funeral home. There is always a funeral program, which has pictures of the deceased and their personal history, including birth and death dates. It often includes a prayer card. There is also a funeral card, which details the order of the service. The funeral can be at either the funeral home or the church. After the burial, there is a meal called the repast, which can be at the church or a restaurant/hall.

Jewish

The Jewish rituals of death and burial are thousands of years old. Since the time of Abraham and Sarah, Jews have dedicated land to cemeteries to bury their loved ones according to Jewish law. The very first established Jewish cemetery is the Cave of Machpelah in Israel, which is the burial cave of our forefathers and foremothers. In many communities, a portion of a local cemetery is often purchased by a synagogue or Jewish organization as the "Jewish Section". Recently, many Jewish cemeteries have set aside sections for interfaith couples and cremation burial.

Jewish burial and memorial practices can and do bring comfort to families because they are prescribed and therefore, serve as a guide for your family as they grieve.

Mourning and Grieving

Grieving is a very personal experience. As you write out your instructions to your children and spouse, explain that you understand each person will deal with your death in their own way and that you hope that each child will respect the others' choices and not call them on it and make an issue.

Faiths and cultures around the world have their own ancient rituals of mourning, which you can explain to your family as they apply to your life.

Two customary Jewish mourning practices are "sitting shiva" and "saying Kaddish." *Shiva*—this word comes from the Hebrew word *shev*, which is the root word for sit and seven. The Jewish mourning period begins immediately after the burial when the family "sits shiva" traditionally for seven days. Friends and relatives come to comfort the mourners and participate in the services when Kaddish is recited. Kaddish is the prayer that mourners recite during the daily service.

One child may choose to sit shiva for a number of days, while another may choose not to stay for all. One child may choose to go to minyan for eleven months; another child may only want to go on Shabbat morning; another may not ever want to say Kaddish. These differences within a family can be hard but give your permission to each person that whatever they choose is all right with you even though it might just about finish you off saying so! By saying so, you are loving them as they are, not as you want them to be. Your permission will go a long way to helping your family, no matter what age, grieve and love *and* be able to deal with others who do their grieving differently.

Sitting shiva—Do you want your family to sit shiva or not? This is a personal choice even though it is certainly customary. Do you want your family to sit for all seven days or are one, two or three days all right with you? In today's world, where children live all over the globe, this is worth thinking about ahead of time, so it won't be a bone of contention between family members if some choose to go home after a few days. Your wishes about sitting shiva are important to your family. Make your wishes known.

Saying Kaddish—A child over 13 years of age customarily says Kaddish for their parents for eleven months and a day. For a sister, brother, wife, husband, son or daughter, tradition calls for thirty days. In today's world, everyone's choice is different. If it matters greatly to you, say so. Write out your wishes for your family's participation in saying Kaddish.

Envelope #2

Preparing This Envelope

Write on the outside of this envelope:

#2
Open Immediately After the Funeral

 This envelope is the tough one. It contains your thoughts on what you want your family to do with your belongings. Hopefully, you have already created a will and a trust and updated them every five years because estate laws frequently change. The work you put into those documents will guide you as you work through the questions that follow. The work you do to complete Envelope #2 can be useful to creating or updating your will and trust documents to reflect your wishes. Be sure to put the date you're writing these instructions on each page. You may find, as time goes by, you are adjusting your decisions. ***Be sure to date any changes.***

Your surviving spouse or partner

 What you put in Envelope #2 depends a great deal on whether you are survived by a spouse or partner. Hopefully, you have determined through your will and trust where your finances and property will be transferred.

No one wants to imagine their spouse living alone after their death; but for many this is the reality for the surviving family. It is important to keep two things in mind as you make decisions for the future: What the survivor wants and is capable of—and their safety. These two things don't always mesh.

This is the time for you to sit down and talk with your inner circle about what could and should happen when either of you is widowed. Your directives to your children will have more strength when you make these decisions while you are both well and of sound mind.

There are so many factors to consider! Key considerations for the surviving spouse might include:

- Where do you want to live?
- Where can you afford to live?
- Who is available to "watch" over you as you live alone—do you have a willing child in the area?
- Do you need medical help?
- Do you need transportation help?
- Is food choice an issue, such as the availability of kosher food?

This also can be tough for children because not everyone lives near their parent and isn't always up to date on the surviving parent's capabilities and needs. Of course, finances play a major part in these decisions also.

These decisions require research, consultation and planning that is best done **before** a spouse is left alone. Of course, circumstances change as time goes by, but having a plan in place can help with transitions. The perfect time to do this is **before** medical needs create an emergency. Make your thoughts known on paper, so your inner circle has a guide to help their living parent navigate living alone.

List your thoughts and preferences on the care of your surviving loved one with a mind to your available resources.

Your belongings

Think carefully about who you want to receive belongings from your life. If you have one grandfather clock that had been passed down to you—and you have four children—it is incumbent on **you** to make the decision who should have this family heirloom, so your children won't fight about it and forever have hard feelings toward each other. Making these choices for them is the hardest thing you can do because each child, regardless of age, has memories that are important to them. Find out *now* what matters to each child. There is no guarantee that they still won't find a way to fight about that clock, but you can help by making the decision for them. That way, they will be mad at you and not each other—and best of all you're not there to fight with!

As you assign these important items to your loved ones, you might consider adding a note at the bottom of that list that, if your family wishes to trade among themselves what you named for them, it's all right. You want them to be happy with their memories, not filled with contention. There is no guarantee this will make everyone happy, but that is not your problem, it's theirs. **You** choose what you want each person to have and let that comfort you.

As another option for family members who may not want the items you've designated for them, give them permission to sell or give away those items. Furniture, jewelry, art, silver and fine china are all beautiful and may be an important part of your children's memories. But today so many of our children—married with families or not—do not live the same lifestyle you did. Giving your permission to sell or donate these items makes it so much easier on them to manage their guilt about not keeping things that were important to you. I know this may hurt deep inside of you, but that is reality. I also suggest taking pictures of treasured family items and making multiple copies for your children. Put a copy for each of them in your envelope and tell your children it's all right to let them go. This is so hard, but I know your children will appreciate your permission.

Money

As new parents, we were over the moon about this gorgeous child now in our lives. As the years go by, not every child fulfills the parents' dreams for them. That does not change the fact that these are your children and you love them. So how do you make everything "fair" or equitable when it comes to giving instructions of how to divide belongings and money?

I cannot tell you what is fair or equitable for you and your family. I can tell you that this takes a tremendous amount of self-examination. The money that is in your accounts is what you've worked a lifetime to accumulate. Only *you* are entitled to make the decision of how it's distributed after your death.

Money is the biggest bone of contention among siblings who feel that they have done more for their parents than another child, therefore they are entitled to more money. I suggest that you carefully think out your approach to distributing your financial assets and take time to rethink it, which could include reviewing your questions and choices with your legal and financial advisors.

There is no guarantee your children will like your decision, but again, it's your money that you accumulated in your lifetime and, therefore, your decision. No question, this is the most difficult thing to do but you should do it for your peace of mind. Whatever you decide—remember, this is **your** decision.

- Make a list of your financial assets and who you want them to go to. Be sure to include the name and contact information of the institution, account numbers and maturity dates of these funds. This should be in conjunction with what you have written in your will and trust documents.

- Consider who you want to add to your accounts and when you wish to do so. Take time now to consult with your financial advisors and financial institutions about the best way to provide your family with this information.

Home, business and vehicles

Whether you are living in a house, a condo or a co-op, tell your children what you want them to do with it after your death. Let them know whether you want them to sell it (and what to do with any proceeds from the sale), whether to donate it to a charity, whether it will go to one of your children or all of them.

There are lots of options to think about!

- Write down what you want your family to do with your home after your death. Be sure to include the name and contact information of any institutions with financial or maintenance interests in your home, such as your condo board, mortgagor and contracted home service providers.
- The same thing applies to your business. If you "give" the business to one child, think about how to compensate your other children if you so choose. Write down what you want your family to do with your business interests after your death. Include the contact information for your legal and accounting advisors.
- Write down what you want your family to do with your vehicles after your death. Include the name and contact information of any financial institutions or maintenance providers, such as lessor, car dealership, storage facility or RV park management. You may be leasing your vehicle, which is easy to give back to the dealer. However, prior to turning in the vehicle, get written confirmation that no further payments are due to the leasing company. If you own your vehicle, think about what you want to have done with it. Consider this carefully because you may have more than one child or grandchild who would love to have your vehicle. Make your thoughts known.

In any of these cases, your legal, financial and spiritual advisors can be helpful resources as you consider various ways to do this, so your decision doesn't create contention or unforeseen issues for your children, which it certainly has the potential to do. Remember, you want your children to get along for the rest of their lives, so this decision is important to think about fully and communicate clearly.

Photos and videos

Make a list of your important photos, albums and videos, and who you wish to have them. In this digital era, it's easy to scan pictures and digitize tapes and share them.

In your world and your parents' world, most pictures were in albums. Who gets them? What about the pictures you have of your grandparents and your great-grandparents? Your kids may not even know them. Do they want those framed photos or albums? Should you have the pictures scanned and identify the people in them in digital form? Ask your children what they think. Enlist their help to deal with the pictures and albums. Your children really don't want to throw out those pictures and albums—but if that's all right with you, tell them.

Genealogy and family record

If you have researched your family genealogy, you will want your labor of love to continue to grow as the years go by. List what website or service you use, your user name and your password so your family can add to it as years go by. Remember: Some accounts may be unretrievable if they expire. Consider this a great gift to your family because it is your family history and theirs.

A family record or registry is contained in many family Bibles. This is a precious family treasure. If you are the guardian of the family Bible, determine who you want to inherit it and be the next record keeper. You want to think this out carefully because there is only one family Bible and you may have several family members who would want it. Remember, this is your family history that goes back generations and it is important to each family member.

Make copies of the family registry so it can be shared with all family members.

Jewelry and art

Some parents have heirloom jewelry; some have none. Some have precious works of art worth a great deal; some do not. Regardless of these items' monetary value, there is no doubt sentimental value to some of your pieces for your children.

Make a list of your jewelry and art pieces. You may want to take a picture of or add a label to the bottom of these belongings if their description on the list is unclear, so no one is confused.

Now is the time to find out who loves what and designate that piece to that child. Make it easy for your children by deciding who gets what, with your permission to trade among themselves if they so choose. If that doesn't appeal to you, consider selling those pieces now and dividing the money between your children.

Valuation of belongings such as art, jewelry and household items may become a bone of contention. Do a bit of research now as to values and include the contact information of your consultants. This will give your family a jump off point that you have established for equity when it's time to distribute these items.

Pets

Your pet is a member of your family. Think carefully about who would be willing to take your pet and love it. Be sure, before you name them, you have their permission.

Write down your pet's veterinarian's contact information and important things to know about your pet, such as care and feeding instructions.

Medical

As we go through life, we accumulate doctors! Realizing that not everyone shares every medical appointment and result with your family, it still is important that you keep an updated list of who you are seeing, contact information and the treatment you're following. That way, your designated person can contact them and let them know that you have passed. You may have a long-standing relationship with some of your doctors and they would definitely want to hear from your family.

If you have mail or auto-refill on your prescriptions, you will want to include that information along with the contact information in Envelope #2.

Legal and financial considerations

As I have explained earlier, your envelopes aren't intended to take the place of any legally binding estate documents like wills, powers of attorney, advance healthcare directives and the like. Careful preparation of these legal documents is critical to protecting yourself and your assets before and after your death.

As a complement to these documents, your envelopes will contain helpful details for your inner circle as they carry out the plans you've made in consultation with your trusted legal and financial advisors.

Designating legal representatives

Your legal and financial advisors can be helpful resources as you consider whom you should designate to handle your affairs. This is the time to consider a trustee if you choose not to have your children handle roles like patient advocate, power of attorney and executor of your estate. Remember, this is your personal business, so *you* get to choose who does what. As you make these decisions, you should ask for and receive each person's permission to be the designated handler of your affairs and make their role known as part of your legal estate work.

In Envelope #2, list your legal representatives and their roles in the affairs of your estate as well as their contact information. Once you have legal estate documents in place, it is important to have them reviewed frequently to make sure they're up to date with current laws, which can change frequently. Also, the same is true for consulting with your financial advisor to ensure your plans are informed by the most current financial regulations.

Something important to consider is the person you designate as your legal trustee to handle everything after you die will be spending hours and hours and weeks and months handling the obligations of your estate. This will take a great deal of time and things don't always conclude quickly. Be sure to receive the permission of the person you designate. They will be dedicating so much time to close your estate. Weigh this obligation against the cost of hiring a professional who charges for their services. This could be an estate attorney, CPA, or financial advisor.

Advance healthcare directives

This is important. If you do not have an advance healthcare directive, please speak with your legal advisor, and have this taken care of immediately.

Please remember that any advance healthcare directive needs to be current to ensure they will be accepted by medical facilities should the need arise. It is imperative that your family knows where your advance healthcare directive is located. You should consider sharing a copy of your directive with your loved ones and any legal representative. It is a good idea for you to have your directive close by so that if you need medical attention, you have that paperwork on hand for EMS and emergency room staff. Especially if you are entering a hospital through an ER, healthcare workers will need to see your directive if you want to avoid any extreme measures they might take.

Insurance policies

If you have insurance policies in place (e.g., life, term, home, vehicle, jewelry, business), you may be surprised to learn that many of these policies are not automatically cancelled or paid when the insured dies. Check with each company about what happens after a death. Be sure to include detailed information on any policies that pertain specifically to your death, funeral and burial, so that they can be easily accessed by your family members to pay for immediate expenses.

Make a list of your insurance policies and who has access and who are the beneficiaries. Include the name and contact information of the insurer, account numbers and any key restrictions regarding claims against these policies.

Technology

This is a tough one to determine what is right for you. So many of us keep everything we do on the computer. That's wonderful, up to a point. It's not unusual over the course of time that we change our passwords to various online resources we use.

How do you let your loved ones know? Put your information on a flash drive **as well as in writing in your Two Envelopes**. Tell your inner circle where you have put this information so they can immediately get access. Remember, as life goes on, things change and your feelings about things change. Pick a date once a year to go back and review your Two Envelopes to make changes you feel are necessary.

Red tape: complications you never thought about

Advance planning makes such a positive difference for your family when they are dealing with details after your death. What no one anticipates is what happens when you are ready to close accounts, cash in policies, cancel credit cards and monthly charges such as cable, cell phone, etc. Red tape creates its own nightmare.

To best handle all the potential problems in closing accounts in your loved one's name, plan on having quick access to the following documents:

- Death certificate (remind your family to request multiple copies from the funeral home)
- Birth certificates for you and your spouse
- Marriage license
- Social Security cards for you and your spouse
- Any adoption or divorce papers

Your family may not know where to find these papers—or you may not even have copies of them. If that's the case, this is the time to write to the city of your birth and request a copy of your birth certificate. While this sounds like overkill, gathering those papers now can save you and your family aggravation and time down the road. As you deal with different institutions, you'll need to make copies of those documents. You don't know what each institution/business will ask for by way of documentation and having these documents close at hand will make things easier for you. Know in advance that you will spending a great deal of time dealing with each institution and it will be incumbent on you to be prepared to give them whatever it is they ask for in order to accomplish your task.

Write a Love Letter

"Before the biblical partner Jacob died, he gathered his family around his bed to bless his family and to say goodbye."

Beresheit (Genesis) Chapter 49

    Writing a love letter to your children and putting it in Envelope #2 is a gift to you and them. This is the perfect opportunity to say whatever you want to your children. These are your children—your babies.

    Let them hear your voice and your memories. Writing your letter (if you're able) rather than typing it gives them a recognizable piece of you. You'll feel better and they will feel all your love.

    This is truly a gift from you to them.

And from Me to You

I wish you peace of mind as you embark on the journey of creating your Two Envelopes. As difficult as this is, after we did our Two Envelopes, my husband and I felt such a sense of relief and comfort.

My hope is you will too.

My best wishes to you for *your* peace of mind,
Rusty Rosenthal Rosman

What to Do with Your Two Envelopes

Writing and filling Two Envelopes is important, but it won't help your family if they cannot find them immediately after your death. You need to put them in a place any of them can find—but no one else would know they are there. This can be quite the quandary. You want them easily accessible but not available to those who have no business looking into them. Think about this carefully. It could be at some point in your life that you need home care. So, you don't want to put these envelopes in your drawers where someone other than your designated person(s) can get them. On the other hand, you don't want to put them in your safety deposit box because the bank may be closed for the weekend or holiday when your designated people need to get to them. Another thing to think about—not every remarriage is smooth with stepchildren and the surviving spouse may not want to give the envelopes to you in a timely manner for your parent's final wishes. So what to do?

A few suggestions and please, keep in mind these are only suggestions. Purchase a fireproof lock box and think about where you want it to reside. Put your envelopes in there and provide the code to your designated responsible person for your arrangements—your children, your funeral representative or possibly a very close friend or family member. Another thought is to send Envelope #1 directly to your designated responsible person or all of your children so they can open it as soon as they learn you have died. That way, your final arrangements can easily move forward.

So what about Envelope #2? It could be in your locked fireproof box or someplace that only your designated responsible person(s) would know to look, such as behind a certain picture in a photo album or in a certain book.

The important thing is to think this over carefully and let your family/designated responsible person know where to find the envelopes. It does you no good to fill the envelopes and no one can find them for months—that's not what you want to happen. Talk this over with your family and your legal representative so you can think this over and make a carefully thought-out decision.

Remember, it is imperative that you keep the contents updated as time goes by. Your envelopes should be easy to open and close—on purpose. I suggest you review these envelopes once a year to see what you may want to adjust or modify. Remember to date each page so it's easy to see that it's the most recent update. Select a date to do this that you will remember, such as New Year's Day.

Please be aware: ***Two Envelopes* does not replace a will and a trust.** Instead, what you put in your Two Envelopes are your personal instructions regarding what is to be done when you die and how to find everything related to your belongings. Unlike your will and trust, which are binding legal documents, *Two Envelopes* is an informational guide only and should NOT be considered legal advice.

Acknowledgments

My first thanks go to my parents of blessed memory, Dorothy S. and Jay M. Rosenthal to whom this book is dedicated. I miss them every day. They gave me the opportunity to participate in their end of life planning and opened my eyes to why this is so important. My parents made it very clear that their stated wishes in their envelopes were separate and apart from their will and their trust.

Their planning made a heart hurting time so much easier to navigate. It also helped us continue to be a family because we didn't fight about how and what to do. We KNEW what they wanted and that's what we did.

Many thanks to Rabbi Joseph H. Krakoff for his wisdom, encouragement and insight. Your depth of understanding of families and your hospice work opened a window for me to see how *Two Envelopes* will help people prepare for the inevitable issues after the death of their loved one. And thanks too, for guiding me to David Crumm, publisher of Front Edge Publishing and Susan Stitt, director of marketing at Front Edge Publishing. So many thanks to Daniel E. Harold, who shared his wise experience and legal advice with me. Best lunch companion ever! Many thanks to Lisa Walters for her constructive suggestions, which helped me fine tune certain sections of Envelope #2.

Acknowledgments

I'm so grateful for the conversations I've had with numerous funeral directors of all religions: Josh Tobias of the Ira Kaufman Funeral Chapel generously gave of his time to educate me on family dynamics on funeral arrangements as well as helping me meet funeral directors whose clientele cover many different religious beliefs and practices. Paddy Lynch of Lynch and Sons Funeral Homes, Sarah Brown-Derbah of Haley Funeral Directors, Helon Rahman of Rahman Funeral Home, Stephen Kemp of Kemp Funeral Home and Funeral Director George Grish all gave generously of their time and expertise. I thank them again for teaching me about the religious funeral practices of their clientele.

Stephen M. Rosman, my wonderful husband, encouraged me every step along the way and provided thoughtful insight when I couldn't find the right words. His faith in me kept propelling me forward. My sisters, Joanne Rosenthal Goldstein and Margo Rosenthal Gold, were invaluable guides, excellent sounding boards and amazing proofreaders throughout this writing process. My daughter Lauren Rosman O'Desky and my daughter-in-law Leise Grimmer Rosman were incredible resources, helped me immeasurably with suggestions and proofreading AND they are my best cheerleaders! My son Brian Rosman encouraged me every step of the way and cheered me on. Each and every one of these wonderful people helped enrich this book that you are holding in your hands.

About the Author

Rusty Rosman spent years helping her parents and her in-laws as they aged. Over the years, Rusty saw many of their friends and their families conflicted over final arrangements and family confrontations. After making sure her parents updated their estate planning, Rusty encouraged them to write out their final wishes for their funerals, mourning period and then, what they wanted done with their belongings that weren't covered in their legal documents. Rusty is one of four children. Having her parents put their wishes in writing made the heartbreaking experience of a parent's death much easier for all four of them to navigate—because they had their parents' wishes in writing. From that experience, *Two Envelopes* was born.

As a former teacher and commercial real estate broker, Rusty has had experience working with people of all ages and circumstances. As a lifelong community leader, Rusty has served as president and fundraiser for several nonprofit community organizations. In her community where she has lived her entire life, Rusty is a member of the Zoning Board of Appeals and the Property Tax Board.

Rusty and her husband Stephen are the very proud parents of Lauren O'Desky and Brian Rosman, both of whom work in medical and medical related fields. Their six grandchildren are the delight of their lives.

Reach Out to Rusty

If you would like to connect with Rusty Rosman or have her speak to your organization, please see her website at www.RustyRosman.com or email her at TwoEnvelopesABook@gmail.com. This book is helpful to everyone because everyone comes from a family. Your friends and colleagues will thank you for organizing an opportunity to meet Rusty, whether it be in person or via a Zoom call. Reach out today.

Notes for Your Two Envelopes

Funeral Arrangements

This page is for making notes of your initial thoughts.
As you finalize your thoughts, write them out and put them in Envelope #1.

How will your family reach the people who are important to you?

This page is for making notes of your initial thoughts.
As you finalize your thoughts, write them out and put them in Envelope #1.

Your Name

This page is for making notes of your initial thoughts.
As you finalize your thoughts, write them out and put them in Envelope #1.

What name do you want used by clergy, the death notice, obituary and eulogy?

Pictures of You

This page is for making notes of your initial thoughts.
As you finalize your thoughts, write them out and put them in Envelope #1.

This is the time to ask for help in getting a picture(s) you like ready to go in this envelope. Include the date the picture was taken, if you remember!

Personalizing Your Obituary, Death Notice and Eulogy

This page is for making notes of your initial thoughts.
As you finalize your thoughts, write them out and put them in Envelope #1.

Be sure to spend the time to list the important things discussed in this section of the book.

Mourning and Grieving

This page is for making notes of your initial thoughts.
As you finalize your thoughts, write them out and put them in Envelope #1.

Collect Your Thoughts
for Envelope #2

Your Surviving Spouse or Partner

This page is for making notes of your initial thoughts.
As you finalize your thoughts, write them out and put them in Envelope #2.

Your Belongings

This page is for making notes of your initial thoughts.
As you finalize your thoughts, write them out and put them in Envelope #2.

Money, Home, Business and Vehicles

This page is for making notes of your initial thoughts.
As you finalize your thoughts, write them out and put them in Envelope #2.

Photos, Jewelry and Art

This page is for making notes of your initial thoughts.
As you finalize your thoughts, write them out and put them in Envelope #2.

Pets

This page is for making notes of your initial thoughts.
As you finalize your thoughts, write them out and put them in Envelope #2.

Medical

This page is for making notes of your initial thoughts.
As you finalize your thoughts, write them out and put them in Envelope #2.

Designating Legal Representatives

This page is for making notes of your initial thoughts.
As you finalize your thoughts, write them out and put them in Envelope #2.

This is a reminder to be sure to prepare your advance healthcare directive and provide that to your family and legal representative now.

Insurance Policies

This page is for making notes of your initial thoughts.
As you finalize your thoughts, write them out and put them in Envelope #2.

Technology

This page is for making notes of your initial thoughts.
As you finalize your thoughts, write them out and put them in Envelope #2.

Red Tape: Complications You Never Thought About

This page is for making notes of your initial thoughts.
As you finalize your thoughts, write them out and put them in Envelope #2.

Check off that you have gathered your birth certificate, marriage license, Social Security card, veteran paperwork, adoption or divorce papers—and any other legal papers that may be relevant. If relevant, where are your deed and mortgage papers?

- ☐ Birth certificate
- ☐ Marriage license
- ☐ Social Security card
- ☐ Veteran paperwork
- ☐ Adoption papers
- ☐ Divorce papers
- ☐ Deeds papers
- ☐ Mortgage papers
- ☐ Other:_____
- ☐ Other:_____
- ☐ Other:_____
- ☐ Other:_____

Love Letter

This page is for making notes of your initial thoughts.
As you finalize your thoughts, write them out and put them in Envelope #2.